Fast and easy way to lose weight

By

Jane Allan

Table of Contents

Introduction

Weight loss: Weight loss is a decline in body weight coming about because of one or the other deliberate (diet, work out) or compulsory (sickness) conditions. Most examples of weight loss emerge because of the deficiency of muscle versus fat, yet in instances of outrageous or extreme weight loss, protein and different substances in the body can likewise be exhausted. Weight loss, with regards to medication, wellbeing, or actual wellness, alludes to a decrease of the complete weight, by a mean loss of liquid, muscle to fat ratio (fat tissue), or slender mass (to be specific bone mineral stores, muscle, ligament, and other connective tissue). Weight loss can either happen unexpectedly due to malnourishment or a fundamental infection, or from a cognizant work to work on a genuine or saw overweight or corpulent state. "Unexplained" weight reduction that isn't brought about by decrease in calorific admission or exercise is called cachexia and might be a side effect of a serious ailment. Deliberate weight loss is normally alluded to as thinning.

Weight loss is characterized as the decrease in weight and muscle versus fat. Nonetheless, outrageous cases may likewise include loss of protein, lean mass, and different substrates in the body. It might either be deliberate, similar to when you quit eating junk food or unexpected, when it is optional to an illness like contamination or malignant growth.

Weight loss is characterized as the decrease in weight and muscle versus fat. Nonetheless, outrageous cases may likewise include loss of protein, lean mass, and different substrates in the body. It might either be deliberate, similar to when you start an improved eating routine or unexpected, when it is optional to an illness like contamination or malignant growth.

Causes

Different variables become possibly the most important factor with regards to getting in shape. The essential standard included is that the body weight is affected by how much energy that we use in our day to day exercises and how much energy found in the food that we eat. An individual whose weight doesn't change is in all likelihood consuming similar number of calories as he is taking in. The overabundance calories taken in are put away in the body as fat. Subsequently, for individuals who need to get thinner, they can either diminish how much food admission or increment how much energy they consume in their proactive tasks.

Deliberate weight reduction is generally completed to work on an individual's wellbeing and advance wellness.

Individuals who are stout or overweight can benefit fundamentally with this type of weight reduction, as wellbeing dangers can be diminished and sicknesses, like hypertension and diabetes, can be forestalled. Patients who deliberately need to shed pounds can do as such with way of life change systems, predominantly a blend of a low-calorie diet and expanded exercise or movement. Different strategies to get thinner incorporate the utilization of specific drugs. For patients who are seriously corpulent, bariatric medical procedure can be performed to diminish the size of the stomach.

Then again, unexpected weight loss could be a sign of various ailments. Ailments will generally expand the metabolic requests of the body, even in the resting state. Simultaneously, illnesses can prompt a deficiency of hunger or a failure to eat, coming about in diminished caloric
consumption. Beside these, certain sicknesses that influence the gastrointestinal framework can bring about issues in assimilation or retention of supplements. Likewise, exorbitant misfortunes of calories and supplements may likewise happen, particularly in patients with ongoing loose bowels or regurgitating.

A few instances of sicknesses that cause weight loss incorporate lack of healthy sustenance, ongoing contamination, for example, tuberculosis and HIV, well established ailments like hyperthyroidism or Parkinson's illness, various types of malignant growth, and constant sorrow. Stomach related framework conditions prompting weight loss incorporate parasitic diseases coming about in constant [diarrhea, fiery gut disorder or persistent pancreatitis, among others. Stomas or enter cutaneous fistulae can likewise prompt weight loss because of unreasonable loss of supplements. A few meds, explicitly diabetes and chemotherapeutic medications, may likewise incite weight loss.

Proceeded and moderate weight loss can bring about ailment known as squandering or cachexia. This state is related with unfortunate results. With this condition, patients can get in shape in any event, when they are getting an adequate number of calories. Extreme weight reduction can influence different frameworks of the body and could bring about wrecking results, including debilitated mending and resistant reaction, debilitated muscle strength, kidney brokenness, and even demise. Weight lose can be disturbing assuming it happens excessively quick. To get thinner, losing a normal of 1 kg a week is ideal. Any other way, you could wind up losing fit muscle rather than muscle to fat ratio. Individuals who lose more than 5 to 10% of their typical body weight in a range of a year or less for not a great explanation by any means, are encouraged to look for clinical consideration. It is likewise prescribed to counsel a doctor in the event that you experience different side effects, like persistent hack or the runs, along with weight reduction.

Chapter 1

Figure out your body

"Furthermore, I shared with my body, delicately: "I need to be your companion." It took a long breath and answered: "I have been hanging tight for what seems like forever for this".

If you have any desire to be intellectually, inwardly, truly, and profoundly solid beginning by get to know your body.

"Your body is the piece of the Universe you've been given".

Your body is your house; it's your sanctuary. It should be treated with thoughtfulness, apperception and mindfulness. YOU merit your own thoughtfulness, appreciation, and mindfulness.

When was the last time you halted and asked what your body needs?

When did you last feel into your entire body?

Truly said thanks to all your body parts and listened eagerly to your own heart beat? A large portion of us, particularly in the event that we distinguish as female, have a confounded relationship with our bodies regardless of our weight or body type. As a rule we take part in a full out battle with it - the weapons being judgment, analysis, and even disdain. A few of us continually wish our bodies were unique, regardless of our body weight or on the other hand in the event that we're as of now at a solid weight. Or on the other hand we live in a ceaseless condition of detachment from our own bodies, and this makes a constant condition of pressure and dis-ease inside us. We can't carry on with a completely present and mindful life on the off chance that we're at battle with what our identity is. We can't encounter a completely solid and sound body and brilliant in general wellbeing in the event that we're inside whipping ourselves.

What's more, sadly, the world we live in programs us for this steady internal conflict from right off the bat. Society is manipulated to attack our confidence continually. We're instructed to fixate on weight reduction, muscle versus fat, and weight list. On the off chance that you recognize as a female you're probably increasing active work, slimming down, and consuming less calories to keep away from weight gain and lower fat mass. On the off chance that you recognize as a male you're probably centered around power lifting to acquire bulk and accomplish lean muscles. The general message we're taken care of through promotions, media, and television is: In the event that you don't look a specific way you're sufficiently not. Yet, we can battle this programming and wake up to understand that it's all BS and intended to keep us debilitated so we continue consuming and burning through cash in an energy to "be sufficient."

We've been given an exceptional gift. Out of the multitude of spots in the universe that we have investigated, we have never gone over much else heavenly than a human body; nothing more wondrous than the human mind inside that body, and nothing more brilliant than the human energy or soul vitalizing that cerebrum and body.

I went through the majority of my time on earth underestimating its capacities until my side effects started. That was a reminder that shook me conscious and constrained me to restore a profound, careful association with the trillions of cells that make up me. It frequently takes some kind of challenge or wellbeing alarm to shake us cognizant and alert.

That is one of the gifts that dis-slide brings into our lives. Tension can likewise make a separation that keeps us from truly feeling our bodies, truly being in our bodies. The unremitting mental clamor and the stressing and the fear keeps us caught in a circle where we could disassociate with our own vessel. Yet, how might we encounter genuine wellbeing, health, and essentialness on the off chance that we don't treat our body with the regard and love it merits? How might we anticipate that our body should show up for ourselves and capability appropriately in the event that we fail to see how it functions and what it needs to work well as well as to flourish and assist us with flourishing thusly? We can't do extraordinary things in a frail, wiped out body. We can't be all that we want to be in a body that is battling to keep up.

Imagine a scenario in which, rather than seeing your side effects of both tension and stomach issues as discipline, you saw them as security.

It is through our real side effects and absence of health that our body, in the entirety of its insight, addresses us and speaks with us, guides us. In any case, do we tune in? Is it true that we are thoughtful to ourselves, body included? The body is an astute data handling machine that can work delightfully voluntarily. The body keeps the Laws of Nature and is continuously looking for equilibrium or homeostasis. The body is wired for flexibility and can recharge and recover itself under sufficient and ideal circumstances. The body is an impression of our inward world - our considerations, feelings, and natural apprehensions/responsibility/injuries.

Chapter 2

12 Sound Tips on quick and simple method for getting slimmer

1.   Do not skip breakfast

Skipping breakfast won't assist you with getting thinner. You could pass up fundamental supplements and you might wind up eating more over the course of the day since you feel hungry.

The group observed that the absolute everyday energy admission was higher in individuals who had breakfast than in the people who skipped it. By and large, 0.44 kilograms (0.97 pounds) lighter. A few preliminaries zeroed in on the impacts of one or the other having or skipping breakfast and any progressions to body weight. From now onward, indefinitely quite a while, the agreement has been that individuals who have breakfast will more often than not be more slender, and that morning meal eating assists individuals with consuming less calories later in the day, in this manner prompting weight reduction. All the more in this way, Having breakfast might get you on target to settle on sound decisions day in and day out. Individuals who have breakfast will generally be more aware of their weight control plans. More energy. A sound breakfast refuels your body and renews the glycogen stores that supply your muscles with quick energy.

5 Motivations to Have Breakfast

#1: Convenient solution of Fundamental Supplements.

#2: Forestall Weight Gain.

#3: Solid Skin.

#4: Power Your Cerebrum.

#5: Jolt of energy.

2.   Eat customary feasts

Eating at customary times during the day helps consume calories at a quicker rate. It additionally lessens the compulsion to nibble on food sources high in fat and sugar.

Customary feasts happen consistently, normally a few times each day. Exceptional feasts are normally held related to such events as birthday celebrations, weddings, commemorations, and occasions. A dinner is unique in relation to a nibble in that feasts are for the most part bigger, more differed, and more filling than snacks.

Our bodies are modified to detect an absence of food as starvation. At the point when we skip feasts, our calorie torch rate eases back, and that implies less calories consumed over the long run. At the point when you don't eat standard dinners, your torch rate will frequently ease back making it harder to get thinner.

3.   Eat a lot of foods grown from the ground

Foods grown from the ground are low in calories and fat, and high in fiber - 3 fundamental elements for effective weight reduction. They likewise contain a lot of nutrients and minerals.
Products of the soil That Assist with consuming Fat Pitted natural products. It might sound unrealistic, yet peaches are assisting you with battling weight related infections.
Grapefruit.
Kale, spinach, and Swiss chard.
Blueberries.
Cruciferous veggies.
Hot peppers.
Avocado.

The following are 11 of the best natural products to eat for weight reduction.
Grapefruit is a combination of a pomelo and an orange and is generally connected with consuming less calories and weight reduction.

A portion of a grapefruit contains only 39 calories however gives 65% of the reference everyday admission (RDI) for of L-ascorbic acid. Red assortments likewise give 28% of the RDI to vitamin A.

Likewise, grapefruit has a low glycemic file (GI), and that implies it discharges sugar into your circulation system all the more leisurely. A low-GI diet might help weight reduction and weight upkeep, however proof is restricted.

In a concentrate in 85 fat individuals, eating grapefruit or drinking grapefruit juice before feasts for a long time brought about a decline in calorie consumption, a 7.1% reduction in body weight, and further developed cholesterol levels. Furthermore, a new survey found that grapefruit utilization decreased muscle versus fat, midsection circuit, and circulatory strain contrasted with control gatherings.

Organic product is nature's instant bite loaded with nutrients, fiber, and different supplements that help a sound eating regimen.

Natural product is likewise commonly low in calories and high in fiber, which might assist you with getting more fit.

As a matter of fact, eating natural product is connected to a lower body weight and a lower hazard of diabetes, hypertension, malignant growth, and coronary illness.

The following are 11 of the best natural products to eat for weight reduction.

1. Grapefruit

Grapefruit is a combination of a pomelo and an orange and is ordinarily connected with counting calories and weight reduction.

A portion of a grapefruit contains only 39 calories however gives 65% of the reference everyday admission (RDI) for of L-ascorbic acid. Red assortments likewise give 28% of the RDI to vitamin A (1Trusted Source).

Furthermore, grapefruit has a low glycemic record (GI), and that implies it discharges sugar into your circulatory system all the more leisurely. A low-GI diet might help weight reduction and weight upkeep, however proof is restricted (2, 3Trusted Source, 4Trusted Source, 5Trusted Source).

In a concentrate in 85 stout individuals, eating grapefruit or drinking grapefruit juice before dinners for quite some time brought about a lessening in calorie consumption, a 7.1% reduction in body weight, and further developed cholesterol levels (6Trusted Source).

Moreover, a new survey found that grapefruit utilization decreased muscle to fat ratio, midriff circuit, and pulse contrasted with control gatherings (7Trusted Source).

While grapefruit can be eaten all alone, it likewise makes
an incredible expansion to plates of mixed greens and
different dishes.

Synopsis Grapefruit is exceptionally low
in calories and high in nutrients An and C. It could be a
sound nibble before fundamental
dinners to assist with diminishing your general food
consumption.
While grapefruit can be eaten all alone, it likewise makes
an extraordinary expansion to servings of mixed greens
and different dishes.

2. Apples
Apples are low in calories and high in fiber, with 116
calories and 5.4 grams of fiber per enormous organic
product (223 grams)

They have likewise been found to help weight reduction.

In one review, ladies were given three apples, three
pears, or three oat treats — with a similar calorie esteem
— each day for a very long time. The apple bunch shed
2 pounds (0.91 kg) and the pear bunch 1.6 pounds (0.84
kg), while the oat gathering's weight didn't change.
Furthermore, an observational concentrate in 124,086
people established that individuals who ate apples lost a

normal of 1.24 pounds (0.56 kg) per day to day serving north of a four-year time span .

Since low-calorie organic products like apples are really filling, you might eat less of different food varieties over the span of the day. Eminently, an apple is very nearly multiple times as filling as a chocolate bar.

Research shows that apples are best eaten entire — instead of squeezed — to lessen craving and control hunger.

All things considered, two examinations connect squeezed apple to decreases in muscle to fat ratio contrasted with a control drink with similar number of calories. Apple polyphenol remove — produced using one of the organic product's regular mixtures — has additionally been connected to diminished cholesterol levels.

Apples can be delighted in various ways both cooked and crude. Have a go at adding them to hot and cold cereals, yogurt, stews, and mixed greens, or baking them all alone

4.	Berries

Berries are low-calorie supplement forces to be reckoned with.

For instance, a ½ cup (74 grams) of blueberries contains only 42 calories yet gives 12% of the RDI to L-ascorbic acid and manganese, as well as 18% for vitamin K.

One cup (152 grams) of strawberries contains under 50 calories and gives 3 grams of dietary fiber, as well as 150% of the RDI for L-ascorbic acid and practically 30% for manganese.

Berries have likewise been demonstrated to fill. One little investigation discovered that individuals given a 65-calorie berry nibble ate less food at a resulting dinner than those given candy with similar number of calories.

Moreover, eating berries might assist with diminishing cholesterol levels, lessen circulatory strain, and lower irritation, which might be especially useful to individuals who are overweight.

Both new or frozen berries can be added to grain or yogurt for breakfast, mixed in a solid smoothie, blended into heated products, or prepared in a serving of mixed greens.

4.   Stone Organic products
Stone natural products, otherwise called drupes, are a gathering of occasional organic products with a plump

outside and a stone, or pit, within. They incorporate peaches, nectarines, plums, cherries, and apricots.

Stone organic products are low-GI, low-calorie, and plentiful in supplements like nutrients C and A — which make them extraordinary for individuals attempting to shed pounds.

For instance, one medium peach (150 grams) contains 58 calories, while 1 cup (130 grams) of cherries gives 87 calories, and two little plums (120 grams) or four apricots (140 grams) have only 60 calories. Contrasted with undesirable nibble food varieties like chips or treats, stone natural products are a more supplement thick, filling choice.

Stone natural products can be eaten new, slashed up in natural product servings of mixed greens, blended into a generous porridge, or even barbecued or added to flavorful dishes like stews.

5.   Passion Organic product
Enthusiasm natural product, which starts in South America, develops on a wonderful, blossoming plant. It has an extreme external skin — purple or yellow in variety — with a consumable, thick seed mass inside.

One natural product (18 grams) contains only 17 calories and is a rich wellspring of fiber, L-ascorbic acid, vitamin A, iron, and potassium.

For such a little organic product, energy natural product holds more than adequate dietary fiber. As a matter of fact, five of them give 42% of the RDI for less than 100 calories .

Fiber dials back your absorption, assisting you with feeling more full for longer and controlling your hunger.

Moreover, energy natural product seeds give piceatannol, a substance connected to decreases in circulatory strain and further developed insulin responsiveness in overweight men. Notwithstanding, more examination is required .

For weight reduction, enthusiasm natural product is best consumed entirety. It very well may be eaten alone, utilized as a fixing or filling for pastries, or added to drinks.

6.   Rhubarb
Rhubarb is really a vegetable, yet in Europe and North America, it is in many cases arranged like a natural product.

While it has just 11 calories for each tail, it actually packs right around 1 gram of fiber and practically 20% of the RDI for vitamin K.

Moreover, rhubarb fiber might assist with lessening elevated cholesterol, which is a typical issue for individuals who battle with their weight.

In a concentrate in 83 individuals with atherosclerosis — an illness of the courses — those given 23 mg of dried rhubarb separate per pound of body weight (50 mg for every kg) for a considerable length of time encountered a critical reduction in cholesterol and further developed vein capability.

Rhubarb stalks can be stewed and presented with porridge or your number one cereal. In spite of the fact that it tends to be utilized in numerous ways, remembering for treats, it's ideal to adhere to low-sugar rhubarb dishes while attempting to shed pounds.

7.   Kiwifruit

Kiwifruits are little, earthy colored natural products with radiant green or yellow tissue and minuscule dark seeds.

Extremely supplement thick, kiwis are an astounding wellspring of L-ascorbic acid, vitamin E, folate, and fiber, and have critical medical advantages.

In one review, 41 individuals with pre-diabetes ate two
brilliant kiwis each day for a very long time. They
encountered higher L-ascorbic acid levels, a decrease in
pulse, and a 1.2-inch (3.1-cm) decrease in midsection
periphery.
Extra investigations note that kiwi can assist with
controlling glucose, further develop cholesterol, and
backing stomach wellbeing — all extra weight reduction
benefits.

Kiwis have a low GI, so while they truly do contain
sugar, it is delivered all the more leisurely — bringing
about more modest glucose spikes.

Moreover, kiwis are wealthy in dietary fiber. One little,
stripped natural product (69 grams) has more than 2
grams of fiber, while the skin alone gives an additional 1
gram of fiber.

Eats less carbs high in fiber from products of the soil
have been displayed to advance weight reduction,
increment completion and further develop stomach
wellbeing (33Trusted Source). Kiwifruit is delicate,
sweet, and delectable when eaten crude, stripped, or
unpeeled. It can likewise be squeezed, utilized in plates
of mixed greens, added to your morning cereal, or
utilized in heated merchandise.

8.   Melons

Melons are low in calories and have a high water content, which makes them very weight reduction well disposed.

Only 1 cup (150 — 160 grams) of melon, like honeydew or watermelon, gives an unassuming 46 — 61 calories.

However low in calories, melons are plentiful in fiber, potassium, and cancer prevention agents, like L-ascorbic acid, beta-carotene, and lycopene.

Besides, polishing off natural products with high water content might assist you with shedding additional weight.

In any case, watermelon has a high GI, so segment control is significant.

Melons can be delighted in new, cubed, or balled to brighten up a natural product salad. They're additionally effortlessly mixed into natural product smoothies or frozen into natural product popsicles.

9.   Oranges

Like all citrus natural products, oranges are low in calories while high in L-ascorbic acid and fiber. They are additionally very filling.

As a matter of fact, oranges are multiple times more filling than a croissant and two times as filling as a muesli bar.

While many individuals polish off squeezed orange rather than orange cuts, investigations have discovered that eating entire organic products — as opposed to drinking natural product juices — not just outcomes in less yearning and calorie admission yet in addition expanded sensations of completion.
Along these lines, assuming that you are attempting to get thinner, it could be smarter to eat oranges instead of drink squeezed orange. The natural product can be eaten alone or added to your #1 plate of mixed greens or pastry.

10.   Bananas
While attempting to get in shape, certain individuals keep away from bananas because of their high sugar and calorie content.
Their low to medium GI might assist with controlling insulin levels and manage weight — especially for individuals who have diabetes.

Moreover, one review represented that eating a banana each day decreased both glucose and cholesterol in individuals with elevated cholesterol.

Superior grade, supplement thick, and low-calorie food varieties like bananas are crucial to any solid weight reduction plan.

Bananas can be delighted in all alone as a helpful in a hurry nibble or added either crude or cooked to a wide assortment of dishes.

11.   Avocados
Avocados are a greasy, calorie-thick organic product filled in warm environments.

Around 50% of an avocado (100 grams) contains 160 calories, making it one of the most calorie-thick natural products. A similar sum gives 25% of the RDI to vitamin K and 20% for folate.

Notwithstanding their unhealthy and fat substance, avocados might advance weight reduction.
In one review, 61 overweight individuals ate an eating regimen containing either 200 grams of avocado or 30 grams of different fats (margarine and oils). The two gatherings experienced critical weight reduction,

demonstrating that avocados are a savvy decision for those hoping to get in shape

Different investigations have discovered that eating avocados can build sensations of totality, decline craving, and further develop cholesterol levels.

Moreover, an enormous investigation of American eating designs uncovered that individuals who ate avocados would in general have better weight control plans, a lower chance of metabolic disorder, and lower body loads than individuals who didn't eat them.

Avocados can be utilized as a swap for spread or margarine on bread and toast. You can likewise add them to servings of mixed greens, smoothies, or plunges.

5.   Get more dynamic
Being dynamic is vital to getting in shape and keeping it off. As well as giving bunches of medical advantages, exercise can assist with consuming off the overabundance calories you can't lose through diet alone. Break significant stretches of sitting. Move however much as could reasonably be expected during the day eg, get off the transport early and walk, use the stairwell, use house work to raise your pulse (vacuum to music). You could complete 30 minutes daily in 10-minute explodes. Walk or cycle to places in the natural air.

6.   Drink a lot of water

Individuals once in a while mistake hunger for hunger. You can wind up polishing off additional calories when a glass of water is truly what you want.

Water can be truly useful for weight reduction. It is 100 percent sans calorie, assists you with consuming more calories and may try and stifle your hunger whenever consumed before dinners. The advantages are much more noteworthy when you supplant sweet refreshments with water. It is an extremely simple method for scaling back sugar and calories.

In spite of the fact that it's anything but an enchanted answer for losing stomach fat, water assumes a part in weight reduction. Drinking water is a significant piece of remaining sound. Remaining hydrated is basic assuming that you're attempting to shed pounds since it helps your body capability actually and will assist you with feeling better by and large.

7.   Eat high fiber food sources

Dietary fiber or roughage is the part of plant-inferred food that can't be totally separated by human stomach related proteins. Dietary strands are assorted in substance structure, and can be assembled commonly by their solvency, thickness, and age capacity, which influence how filaments are handled in the body. Food sources containing heaps of fiber can assist with keeping you feeling full, which is ideally suited for getting in shape.

Fiber is just tracked down in food from plants, like products of the soil, oats, wholegrain bread, earthy colored rice and pasta, and beans, peas and lentils.

8 High-Fiber Food varieties That Can Assist You With getting in shape

High-Fiber Grain Cereal. Serving size: ½ cup.
Chia Seeds. Serving size: 1 ounce (2 Tbsp.)
Naval force Beans. Serving size: ½ cup, cooked.
French Green Beans. Serving size: ½ cup, cooked.
Raspberries. Serving size: 1 cup.
Lentils. Serving size: ½ cup, cooked.
Chickpeas.
Blackberries.

8.   Read food names

Knowing how to peruse food names can assist you with picking better choices. Utilize the calorie data to sort out how a specific food squeezes into your day to day calorie stipend on the weight reduction plan.
Step by step instructions to Peruse Food Marks for Weight reduction
Decide the serving size. At the highest point of the nourishment mark, you will find the food's serving size, as well as the quantity of servings contained in each bundle.
Ascertain the calories consumed.

Assess fat, cholesterol, and sodium.
Assess fiber, nutrients, calcium, and iron

9.   Use a more modest plate

Utilizing more modest plates can assist you with eating more modest bits. By utilizing more modest plates and bowls, you might have the option to slowly become acclimated to eating more modest parts without going hungry. It requires around 20 minutes for the stomach to tell the mind it's full, so eat gradually and quit eating before you feel full. Utilizing a more modest plate at feast time will assist with controlling your segments, decrease your calorie admission, and help in your weight reduction achievement. Utilize a more modest plate - Set aside cash. This one simply checks out. On the off chance that you are involving a more modest plate for your dinners, you are eating less and this will assist you with cutting food costs.

In one trial, directed by Brian Wansink from Cornell College and Koert van Ittersum from the Georgia Organization of Innovation, it was found that a shift from 12-inch plates to 10-inch plates brought about a 22% reduction in calories.

10.   Do not boycott food varieties

Prohibit no food sources from your weight reduction plan, particularly the ones you like. Prohibiting food sources will just cause you to long for them more.

There's not a really obvious explanation you can't partake in a periodic treat as long as you stay inside your day to day calorie remittance.

11.   Do not stock low quality food
To keep away from enticement, don't stock low quality food - like chocolate, rolls, crisps and sweet bubbly beverages - at home. All things being equal, choose solid tidbits, for example, natural product, unsalted rice cakes, oat cakes, unsalted or unsweetened popcorn, and natural product juice.

12.   Cut down on liquor
A standard glass of wine can contain however many calories as a piece of chocolate. After some time, drinking a lot of can without much of a stretch add to weight gain.

13.   Plan your dinners
Attempt to design your morning meal, lunch , supper and snacks for the week, ensuring you adhere to your calorie recompense. You might find it supportive to make a week by week shopping list.

Conclusion

A believe with the key words and factors written in this book, you can actually lose wait fast and easily.

www.ingramcontent.com/pod-product-compliance
Lightning Source LLC
Chambersburg PA
CBHW071504150726

48000CB00006B/2693